Catching a Cold

How you get ill, suffer and recover

Steve Parker

FRANKLIN WATTS
New York • London • Toronto • Sydney

Franklin Watts, Inc.
387 Park Avenue South
New York, NY 10016

Library of Congress Cataloging-in-Publication Data

Parker, Steve.
    Catching a cold / by Steve Parker.
        p.   cm. — (Body in action)
    Includes index.
    Summary: Explains what happens to the body when one has a cold,
such as having a fever, sneezing, and coughing. Includes projects.
    ISBN 0-531-14146-2
    1. Cold (Disease)—Juvenile literature.   [1. Cold (Disease)]
I. Title.   II. Series.
RF361.P37   1992
616.2'05—dc20   91-747
                                                                     CIP AC

Printed in Great Britain

Medical consultant:
Dr. Puran Ganeri, MBBS, MRCP, MRCGP, DCH

Series editors: Anita Ganeri and A. Patricia Sechi
Design: K and Co.
Illustrations: Hayward Art
Photography: Chris Fairclough
Typesetting: Lineage Ltd, Watford

The publisher would like to thank Elizabeth and Ann
Leather for appearing in the photographs of this book.

CONTENTS

4 Feeling ill

6 Germ attack

8 The cold takes hold

10 The need for rest

14 Fighting back

17 Battle in the blood

20 Being immune

22 Getting better

25 Complete recovery

27 Staying healthy

28 Things to do

30 Glossary and resources

32 Index

Feeling ill

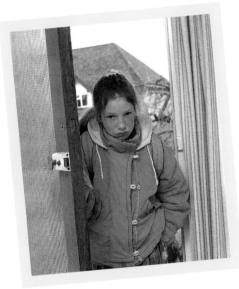

△ You may be coming down with a cold and not realize it. You may feel slightly tired, shivery and dizzy. But you do not yet know that you are ill.

▷ Colds and many other illnesses are caused by tiny germs. Your body's natural defenses usually keep these germs out. But sometimes germs get inside your body, multiply and make you ill.

Most people are well for most of the time. But now and then, illness strikes. It may be something minor, like a common cold, or something more serious, such as measles or even pneumonia. But the human body has great powers of healing and recovery. In many cases, you will probably get better simply by staying at home and resting for a while. At other times, you may need special medical care.

Tear fluid washes dust and many germs from eyes

Sticky **mucus** traps and removes most germs in nose and airways

Hairs in the **nose** filter out many germs from inhaled air

Skin forms a nearly germproof barrier over the body

Acid in **stomach** kills many germs in food

ILLNESS FACTS

- Among the most common illnesses are gum diseases, and the common cold.
- Some illnesses are unusual in one area, but common in another. Malaria is rare in Europe and North America. Yet in the tropical regions shown in dark green on the map, 50 million people catch malaria a year. Up to a million die from it.
- Malaria germs are spread by mosquitoes.

If they suck the blood of a person with malaria, they take in the germs. When they bite another person, the malaria germs may enter their blood.

- The main symptoms of malaria are high fever and weakness.

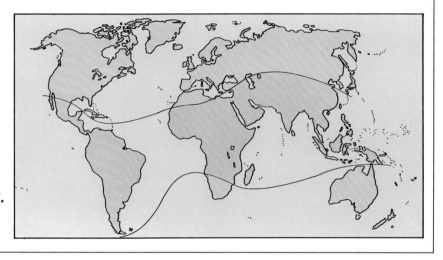

WHEN ARE PEOPLE ILL?

Which illnesses are most common where you live? What time of year do they usually occur? Ask your teacher about your school's attendance records. These show who has been out sick and when. Are more people ill in the summer or the winter? Draw a graph or table of the results of your survey.

Sometimes an illness

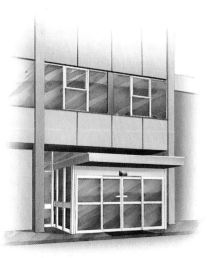

such as "flu" (this is short for influenza) affects so many people that a whole school, office or store may have to be closed. This is called an epidemic. Your doctor or local druggist may have some more information about epidemics of colds, sore throats and flu in your area. (See also page 28 for more ideas.)

Germ attack

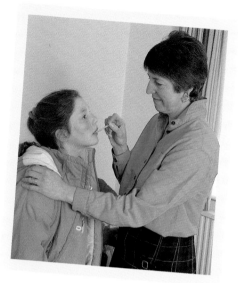

Germs are tiny living things that can cause illnesses, such as colds. Illnesses caused by germs invading the body are called infections. Germs are all around you – in the air, in the soil, and on everyday objects. Normally, your body can resist them. But if there are too many germs, or your body is tired or run-down, the germs more easily multiply and make you ill.

△ A high temperature, or fever, is an early sign of infection. A clinical thermometer is used to take your temperature.

▷ When you are healthy, your temperature stays about the same. It is controlled by a part of your brain called the hypothalamus. This switches on cooling processes, such as sweating, when you get too hot. It turns on warming processes, like shivering, when you get too cold. When you have a cold, your temperature rises as your body starts to fight the cold germs.

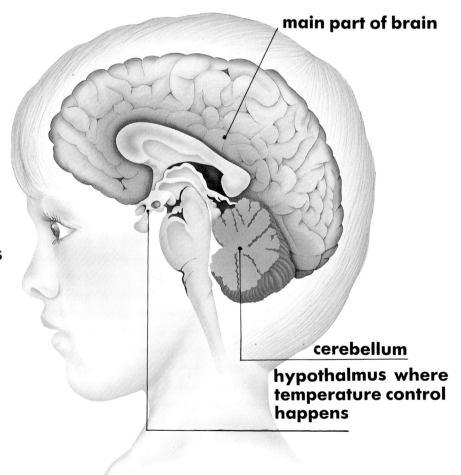

main part of brain

cerebellum

hypothalmus where temperature control happens

TAKING YOUR TEMPERATURE

A clinical thermometer is a sealed glass tube containing mercury, which is poisonous. It must be used with great care. Ask an adult to take your temperature safely and correctly.

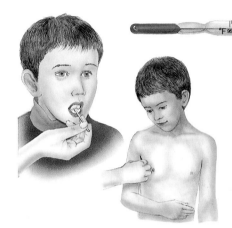

1 Ask an adult to shake the thermometer and place it in your mouth for 5 minutes. For a young child, the thermometer can go under their armpit for a couple of minutes.

2 As your body warms the mercury, it expands along the hole in the glass tube. You can then read how high your temperature is on the scale running along the thermometer's side.

TEMPERATURE FACTS

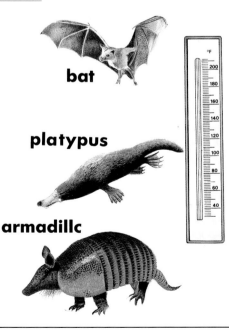

bat

platypus

armadillo

• The human body is "warm-blooded." The temperature inside it stays much the same, unless it is ill.
• Your normal body temperature is about 98.6°F.
• This varies by about 0.5°F as part of your body's daily rhythm. It is lowest in the early morning, at around 2 to 5 a.m.

• Other warm-blooded animals have different body temperatures. A bat's may reach 110°F, a platypus's 90°F and an armadillo's as low as 77°F.
• A fever of 104°F or above can be very dangerous. This is called hyperthermia.
• If your body gets too cool, you may suffer from hypothermia.

The cold takes hold

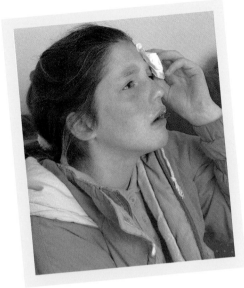

As the germs continue to multiply inside you, your body's natural inner defenses start to fight back. It is fighting back that causes many features of your cold, such as a fever, headache, runny nose, watery eyes, sneezing and coughing. These features are known as symptoms. Each illness has its own particular set of symptoms, which help us to identify it.

△ Sweating is an automatic reaction when your body is too hot. As the watery sweat dries on your skin, it draws heat from your body and cools you down.

▷ As the fever rises, it confuses your body's temperature control. Sometimes you feel hot and sweaty. At other times you feel cold and shivery. When you get cold, tiny muscles pull hairs in your skin upright. This forms goose bumps, or goose pimples.

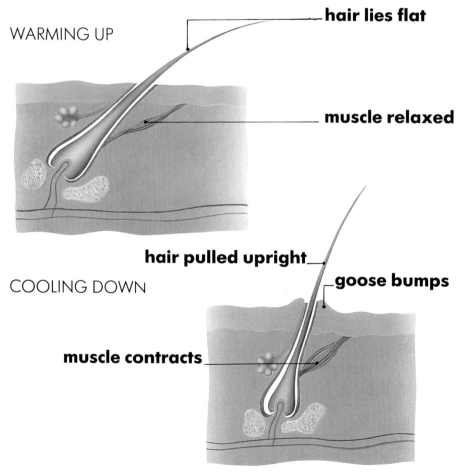

WARMING UP

hair lies flat

muscle relaxed

hair pulled upright

COOLING DOWN

goose bumps

muscle contracts

GERM FACTS

• There are thousands of types of infectious germs. Each one causes a particular type of infection.

• The smallest germs are called viruses. It would take millions to cover a pinhead. They cause colds, measles and chicken pox.

• Bacteria are bigger germs than viruses. Even so, a row of a thousand bacteria would only stretch a millimeter. They cause such illnesses as scarlet fever, whooping cough and diphtheria.

• Tiny fungi can also cause infections, such as ringworm and athlete's foot.

• Protozoans are tiny animals, bigger than bacteria but still too small to see. They cause some types of dysentery and other tropical illnesses.

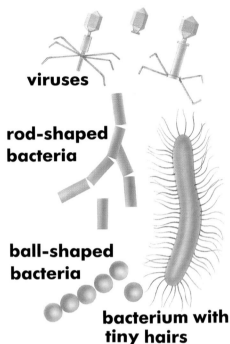

viruses

rod-shaped bacteria

ball-shaped bacteria

bacterium with tiny hairs

TEMPERATURE SURVEY

Your body tries to keep its temperature constant, but it may need help. Clothes are one form of help. In very hot places, people wear loose-fitting robes which shield their bodies from the glare of the sun, yet allow cooling air to flow over the skin. In very cold places, thick, furry clothes keep the body's warmth in. Find out about how different clothes and activities affect your body temperature by asking an adult to take your temperature at various different times. Try this after you have run about in a swim suit on a sunny day, had a warm bath, taken a cold shower, or gone for a walk well wrapped up in warm clothes. Is your temperature always about the same? If it rises or falls slightly, does it soon return to normal?

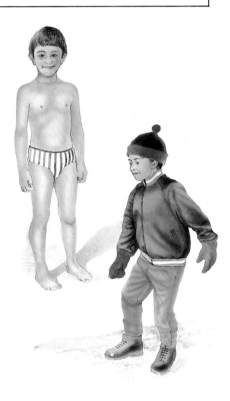

The need for rest

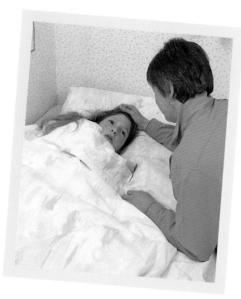

As the cold germs multiply, and your body steps up its fight against them, you become a sort of battleground. You will probably feel tired and in need of a rest. Don't ignore these feelings. They are your body's way of telling you that if you try to stay active, you will use up energy that could be used to fight the germs. Rest and keep warm (but not too hot). Drink plenty of water and juice, to keep up your body's fluid levels.

△ In most cases, it is a good idea to let your body rest while you are ill. Trying to carry on with everyday life could make you feel worse.

▷ The germs that cause a cold mainly affect the linings of your nose and throat. They make them swollen, red, sore and stuffed-up. As part of your body's defense system, the linings produce lots of a sticky substance called mucus.

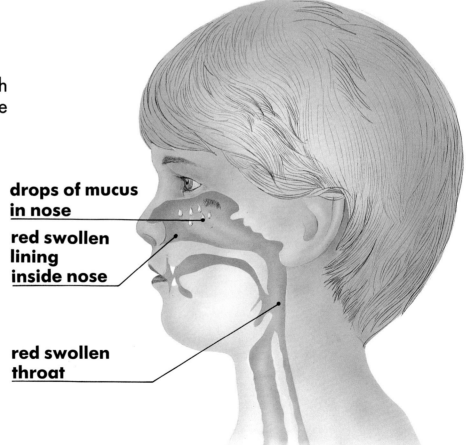

drops of mucus in nose

red swollen lining inside nose

red swollen throat

SNEEZE AND COUGH FACTS

- The swelling and mucus in your nose block your breathing passages. Your body's automatic reaction is to sneeze, to remove the blockage.
- When you sneeze, air blasts out of your nose at 100 miles an hour — as fast as an express train!
- The swelling and mucus in your throat also cause problems. Coughing helps to clear these up.
- When you cough, air rushes past the vocal

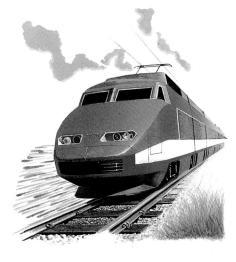

cords in your lower throat, so fast that it sounds like a shot from a gun!
- Coughing and sneezing help to clear your breathing passages. But with a bad cold, they can keep you awake and prevent you from getting enough rest. A spoonful of cough medicine may help to ease a cough so you sleep better.

WHAT'S IN A SNEEZE?

Sneezes spread cold germs. To show how this happens, put a few drops of water, colored with food dye, into the end of a bicycle pump. Blow a "sneeze" from the pump onto a sheet of newspaper about 3 feet away. Then blow one into a nearby tissue. In a real sneeze, the colored spots would be drops of mucus, full of cold germs. A single sneeze can blow 100,000 drops into the air. Other people inhale them and catch a cold themselves. You should always catch a sneeze in a handkerchief.

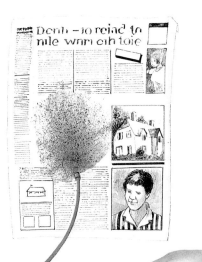

INNER DEFENSES

A main part of your body's defense against illness is your lymph system. This is a network of tubes running through your body. They carry lymph fluid, a pale liquid that contains nutrients and germ-fighting cells. Lymph fluid is made from the liquid part of blood. It seeps out of your small blood vessels into the spaces between your body parts, and flows

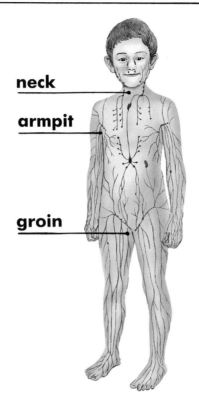

neck

armpit

groin

back through lymph tubes into your blood system in your chest. In certain parts of your body, the lymph tubes widen into clusters of lymph nodes, sometimes called "glands," as shown here. (They are not true glands, since they do not make hormones or digestive chemicals.) Germ-fighting cells are made here and the lymph fluid is cleaned of dead germs.

INSIDE A LYMPH NODE

Lymph fluid flows into a lymph node through small tubes. It usually flows out through one large tube. Valves make sure the fluid flows one way only. The main part of the node is made up of clumps of germ-fighting cells, wrapped in connective tissue. Lymph nodes also have an ordinary blood supply, like the other parts of your body.

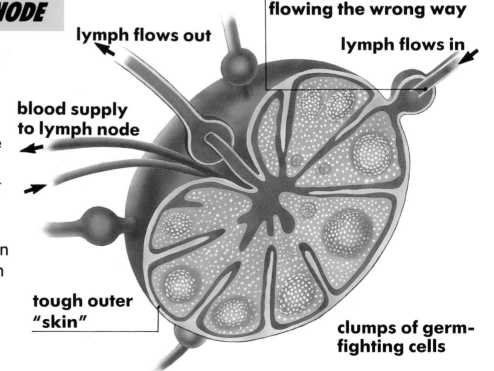

valve prevents lymph from flowing the wrong way

lymph flows out

lymph flows in

blood supply to lymph node

tough outer "skin"

clumps of germ-fighting cells

12

To see how lymph nodes swell and feel hard during an infection, use a balloon and some water from a pitcher and from a cold tap. Blow up the balloon several times first, to make it stretchy and slack. Then half-fill it with water from the pitcher. Notice how the balloon is soft and squishy, and can be prodded easily. This is like a healthy lymph node. Now attach the balloon to the water spout and slowly force in extra water, under pressure. See how the balloon becomes hard and difficult to press in. This is like a lymph node during an infection. It is swollen with extra lymph fluid, germ-fighting cells and dead germs.

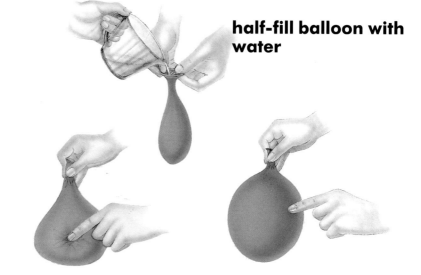

half-fill balloon with water

Half-filled balloon is soft and squashable.

Full balloon is stretched tight and hard.

LYMPH FACTS

• Your heart acts like a pump in your blood system. Your lymph system does not have a pump. It squeezes fluid along using muscles and body movements.

• Every minute, 10 milliliters of lymph flows back into your blood system. This is about the same amount as in two teaspoonsful.

• When an infection such as a cold starts, your lymph system becomes more active. Germ-killing cells gather in the nodes, and extra fluid collects there as germs die. This makes the nodes swell.

• When you are healthy, your larger lymph nodes are bean-shaped and about three-quarters of an inch across.

• When you are ill, the nodes may swell to twice this size, about as big as a table tennis ball. You can see and feel them as swollen lumps under your skin. They are often called "swollen glands." They are very tender and hurt when they are pressed.

Fighting back

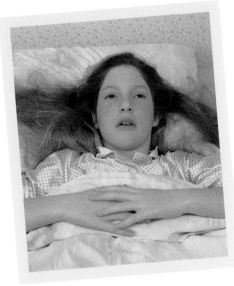

△ As your cold gets worse, you may feel drowsy and fall asleep. This is a natural reaction to many types of illness.

Since the germs that cause a cold mainly affect your nose and throat, this is where the chief symptoms of a cold occur. But they also spread around your body in your blood and lymph systems. Lymph fluid contains many germ-fighting cells, but most of these come originally from your blood. In fact, your blood contains whole armies of cells (the immune system), ready to attack and destroy the invaders. These attackers are called white blood cells. They are not really white, but look jellylike and transparent.

▷ This is what your blood looks like under a microscope. It has two main types of cells. Red cells carry oxygen around your body. White cells help fight disease. Both types of cells float in a pale yellow liquid, called plasma.

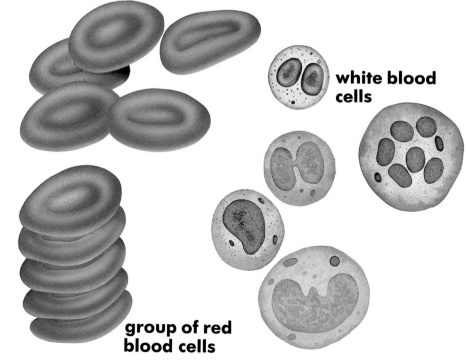

red blood cells

white blood cells

group of red blood cells

BLOOD FACTS

- There are about 5 million red blood cells in a pinhead-sized spot of blood. Each is shaped like a doughnut.
- The same amount of blood contains 5,000 white blood cells.
- The same amount of blood also contains 250,000 pieces of cells, called platelets. They help blood to clot in a wound.
- Some illnesses affect the blood cells. In anemia, the red blood cells cannot carry enough oxygen around the body. This may be because they die too quickly, or are misshapen or faulty.
- People with anemia feel tired and get out of breath easily. They are more at risk of catching other illnesses.
- In a type of anemia, called sickle-cell anemia, the red blood cells are not round but crescent (sickle) shaped. They stick together and block small blood vessels, so they cannot carry oxygen properly.

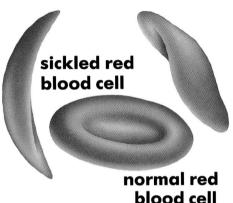

sickled red blood cell

normal red blood cell

MAKE YOUR OWN BLOOD SAMPLE

See how different parts of blood flow around the body by making a model blood sample. Add hot water to a 3-5 inch clear glass jar. Keep adding sugar until all but a few granules have dissolved. This is the plasma. Add leaves from half a used tea bag. The different-sized leaves are the various blood cells and molecules. Stir the water and let it become still. The large leaves, the cells, will sink to the bottom. The smaller leaves, small cells and large molecules, will float in the water. This is what happens when the doctor takes a blood sample and leaves it to stand in a jar. The blood cells sink to the bottom, leaving clear plasma above them. Now swirl the water around, and see how the leaves lift up and flow with it. This is how blood cells are swept along in the blood, around your body.

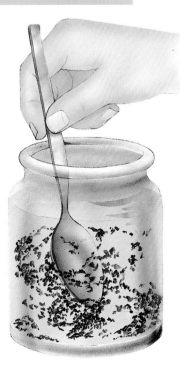

THE GERM-EATERS

White blood cells sometimes squeeze out of your blood and lymph tubes and travel among your body parts, to hunt for germs. There are several main kinds of white blood cells. Some "eat" germs by flowing around them (see below). These cells can live for about 10 days. If they eat hundreds of germs, though, they die sooner than this. Millions of dead white cells and germs

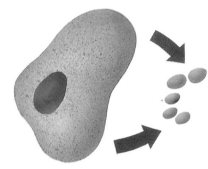

White blood cell flows towards clump of germs.

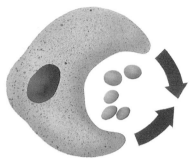

White blood cell flows around germs.

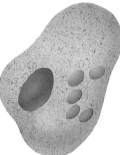

White blood cell engulfs germs and kills them.

make pus, the greenish or yellow fluid formed by infection.

SEE HOW THEY MOVE

Red blood cells are simply swept along by the blood, but white blood cells can move by themselves. They change shape as they ooze along in search of germs. To see how they do this, partly fill a clear plastic bag with water, and tie it firmly at the top. The bag is like the stretchy "skin" around the blood cell. Roll the bag along a table or the floor. See how easily it changes shape as it rolls along.

Battle in the blood

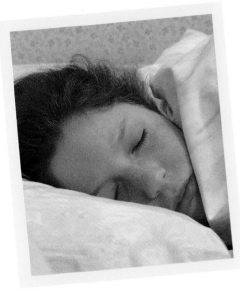

You have billions of white blood cells, but millions die in the fight against infection. Even when you are healthy, old blood cells are dying all the time. To replace them you make new cells, mainly inside your bones.

△ While you sleep, your body has a good chance to use all its fighting power to kill off the cold germs inside it.

▷ Some bones have spaces inside, and are filled with a jellylike substance called bone marrow. In the marrow, special cells are busy multiplying to make new blood cells. These flow into blood vessels running through the marrow, and enter your blood system. The marrow is shown in pink.

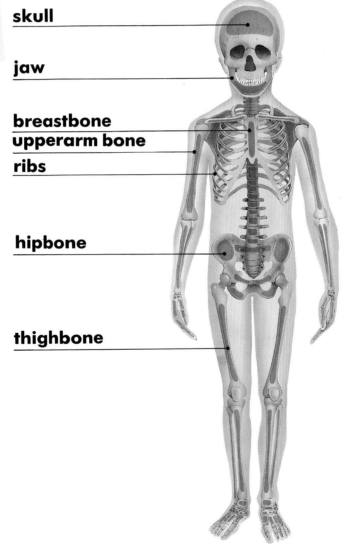

skull

jaw

breastbone
upperarm bone
ribs

hipbone

thighbone

MARROW FACTS

- Marrow makes an amazing 2 million red blood cells a second!
- In an average lifetime, the marrow makes half a ton of red blood cells.
- On average, a red blood cell lives for 3 or 4 months. During this time it makes more than 50,000 trips around the body.
- Many white blood cells are also made in the marrow. Other white cells, called lymphocytes, are made in the lymph nodes.
- A typical white cell can live for several days in a healthy body. When fighting an infection, it lives for only a few hours.
- The bone marrow stores millions of white blood cells. When germs invade the body, the cells swarm into the blood to fight them.
- At the same time, the bone marrow and lymph system step up their production. They make millions of new white blood cells every minute, to defend the body.

LOOKING AT BONE MARROW

Bone marrow is soft and squishy, and could easily get damaged. But it is well protected inside its tough casing of bone. To find out how good this protection is, ask your local butcher or meat supplier to give you a "marrowbone" (the kind given to pet dogs). This is usually an animal bone, sawn through to show the marrow-filled space inside. Meat-eaters such as dogs, wolves, hyenas and jackals have huge

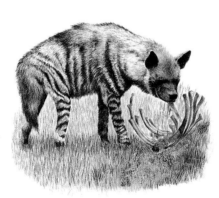

back teeth, to crunch bones open and get to the nutritious marrow. If you want to see more of the marrow, ask an adult to crack the bone open with a hammer. (Wrap it in a cloth first, to catch flying splinters.) See how much force these animals have to use, to get at their meal!

THE SPLEEN

Your spleen is part of your lymph system. It is in your left upper abdomen, just behind your stomach, and is about the size of a clenched fist. Inside the womb, a developing baby's spleen makes white blood cells, like the bone marrow. As the baby is born and grows, the spleen makes fewer and fewer blood cells. In a child and adult, its main jobs are connected with cleaning the blood.

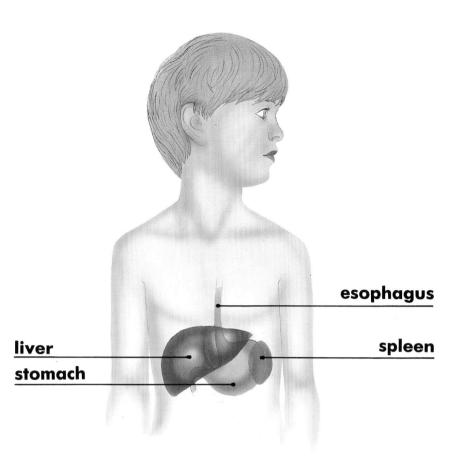

esophagus

liver

spleen

stomach

INSIDE THE SPLEEN

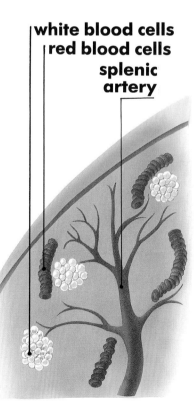

white blood cells
red blood cells
splenic
artery

One of the spleen's main functions is to break down and dispose of old red blood cells. Blood flows into the spleen along a tube called the splenic artery. Inside, some of it flows through clusters of red blood cells. Some red cells are stored here, while old, worn-out cells are taken apart and disposed of. The cells contain iron, a valuable body mineral. It is sent back to the bone marrow for recycling into new red cells. Some of the blood coming into the spleen flows through clumps of white blood cells, which eat germs and other debris and so clean the blood. The spleen also helps to make new lymphocytes, one of the main kinds of white blood cells.

Being immune

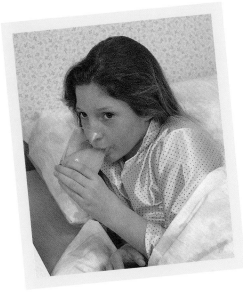

Infections like colds are very common. Some people catch two or three colds every year. But you normally only catch certain infections, such as chicken pox, once in your lifetime. When your body has had this type of infection once, it develops a resistance to it so you do not get it again. This resistance is called immunity. It is produced by your body's immune system.

△ As your body continues to fight against the cold germs, you still need to rest. You also need plenty to drink because the battle uses up lots of fluids and can cause dehydration.

▷ The thymus gland is part of your immune system. It is in your chest, next to the heart. White blood cells called lymphocytes are made in this gland. They are able to recognize invading germs. These lymphocytes enter the lymph system. When germs invade, they "tell" other white blood cells to begin the battle.

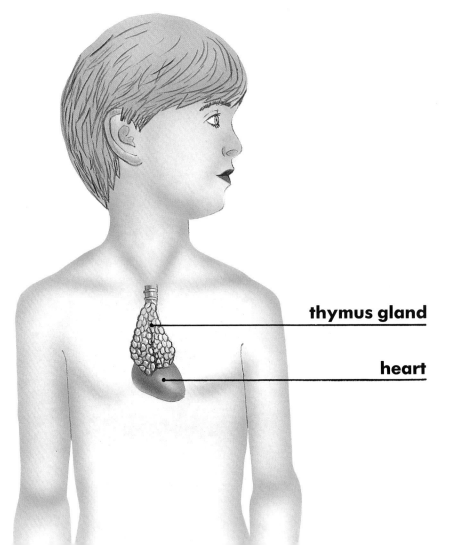

thymus gland

heart

• Immunization is the giving of a vaccine that makes you resistant to an infection, without actually suffering from it.

• The BCG injection gives resistance to tuberculosis. It is usually given a few weeks after birth. It may also be given at about 12 years of age.

• A course of injections given at 2, 3 and 4 months old makes you immune to three serious infections. These are

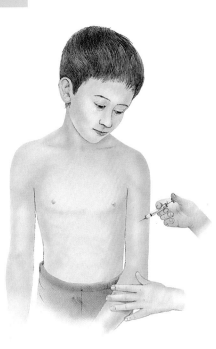

diphtheria, tetanus and whooping cough. The injection is repeated just before you start going to school.

• The polio vaccine gives immunity to polio. Doctors often put the vaccine drops on a lump of sugar to make it taste better.

• For some of these immunizations, you may have "booster" shots when you are older. This ensures long-lasting protection.

ANTIBODIES

During an infection, white blood cells called lymphocytes make substances called antibodies. These are much smaller than even the tiniest germ. They stick onto germs and destroy them. In the middle of an infection, each of the millions of lymphocytes in your blood and lymph fluid makes an amazing

2,000 antibodies every second! A typical antibody is Y-shaped.

Two sticky patches on the ends of the arms of the Y hold on to the germs.

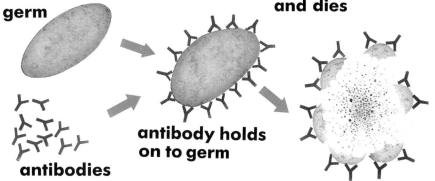

germ

antibodies

antibody holds on to germ

germ bursts open and dies

Getting better

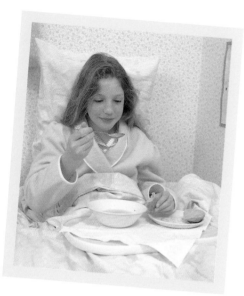

Gradually, your body starts winning the battle against the cold germs. Although you may have had a cold before, there are many types of cold germs (viruses). The antibodies you made against the last type you had might not work against these new ones. This is why you cannot become immune to viral infections such as colds. However, with its white cells, antibodies and other defenses, your body can kill off the new germs.

△ You may not feel like eating when you are very ill. But as you start to recover, you need to build up your strength again. Start by eating small amounts of nutritious, easily-digested food, such as soup.

▷ Some chest infections have symptoms like a cold, but are more serious. The doctor may then arrange for the person to have a chest X-ray. This is a picture of the inside of the chest. It shows whether the lungs or heart are diseased.

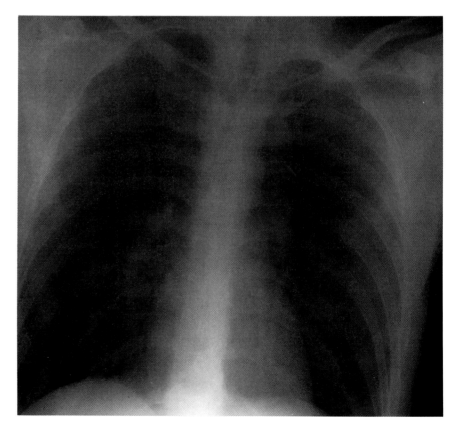

HOW CLEAN IS THE AIR?

Air that is full of dust, dirt and germs is more likely to make you ill than clean air. In some areas, especially large cities, the air is not very clean. You may not be able to see any dirt, but sometimes you can see smog. Put a clean, slightly damp white handkerchief or cloth on a window ledge or clothesline outside. After a few hours, the cloth may be covered with specks of dust and dirt.

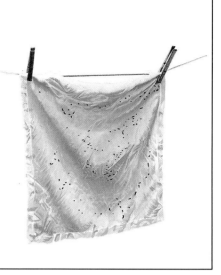

CLEANING THE AIRWAYS

Your body has several defenses against airborne particles (see page 4). The linings of your nose, throat, windpipe and lungs make sticky mucus that traps dust, germs and so on. Some linings also have rows of tiny hairs, called cilia. The cilia sway back and forth, slowly pushing the dirty mucus along, so that you can swallow it or blow it out of your nose.

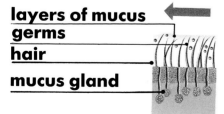

layers of mucus
germs
hair
mucus gland

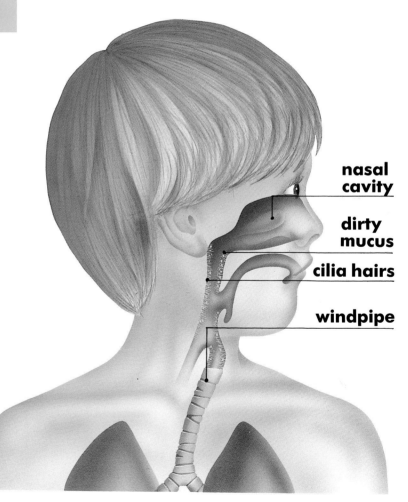

nasal cavity

dirty mucus

cilia hairs

windpipe

SYMPTOM RELIEF

Some illnesses can be gotten rid of, or cured, by medicines. The common cold is not one of them. However, there are things you can do or take to ease the cold symptoms, so that you do not feel quite so ill. Medicines such as acetaminophen help to lower your body temperature so you do not feel feverish. Inhaling warm steam or vapors loosens mucus in your airways so you can breathe more easily.

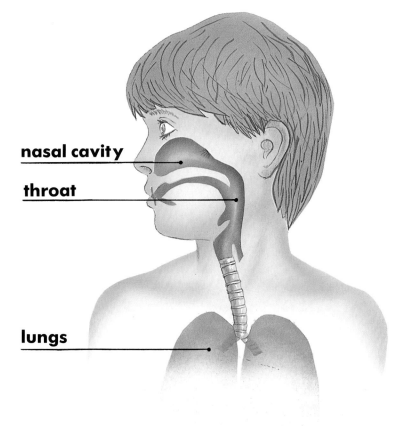

nasal cavity

throat

lungs

HEALTHY FACTS

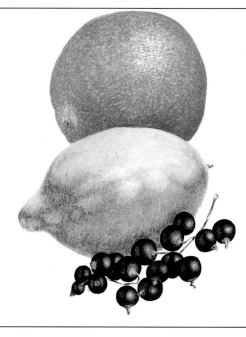

• Substances called vitamins are important for good health. If the foods you eat do not contain enough vitamins, you may fall ill. You can also take vitamin pills.
• Vitamin B is found in fresh vegetables and in liver. It is needed to make healthy red blood cells. Lack of it

can cause anemia.
• Vitamin C is found in many foods, such as oranges, lemons, and other types of fruit. Lack of it causes rough skin, bleeding gums and stiff arms and legs.
• Large amounts of vitamin C may help some people resist colds. But is not a sure way of protection.

Complete recovery

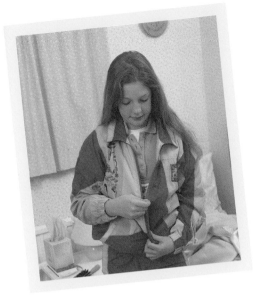

A few days after you first felt unwell, your cold is fading fast. You probably feel much better and want to get out and about again. But be careful at first. Sometimes, trying to get back to normal too quickly can delay your recovery, or even bring the illness back. This is called a relapse. With care and rest, however, the last cold germs are killed off, and the illness is soon gone.

△ Your body's defenses have won the battle, and your health and energy are quickly getting back to normal.

▽ In places such as Europe and North America, we have generally good health. In many areas of the world, people are ill much more often. The illnesses they catch are often serious, like the ones shown below.

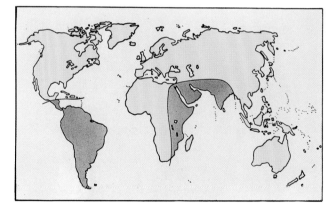

schistosomiasis (infection with a tiny worm) affects the regions shown in dark green

sleeping sickness (trypanosomiasis) affects the regions shown in dark green

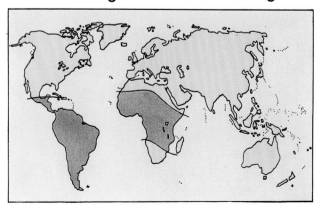

PILLS AND MEDICINES

If you need medical treatment for an illness, the doctor will choose the best type of drug to give you. This is called prescribing the treatment. Some treatments are in the form of pills or tablets, which you swallow. Some treatments are in the form of liquid medicines, which you may sip from a special measuring spoon.

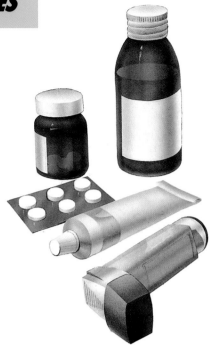

Other treatments come as creams or lotions, which are rubbed on. These are particularly useful for rashes and other skin diseases. Yet other treatments are in the form of a fine spray or mist, which you breathe in from an inhaler. These are especially helpful for people with breathing problems and lung illnesses.

ILLNESS AND CURE FACTS

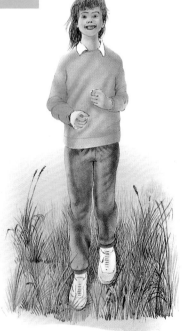

• There are several main kinds of illnesses, apart from infections. In an allergy, for example, your body reacts as if it has been invaded by germs. But the invaders are actually harmless bits of dust or pollen grains from plants.
• Common illnesses caused by allergies are hay fever and asthma.
• Heart disease is another major kind of illness. In Europe and North America it kills one person in four.
• Doctors and scientists are working hard to find a cure for many illnesses, such as cancer and AIDS.
• Immunization was a central part of the worldwide fight against smallpox, a very serious infection. The fight began in 1967, and was so successful that by 1979, the disease had disappeared.

Staying healthy

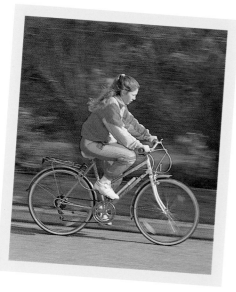

With a cold, your body really cures itself. More serious illnesses may need medical help. Doctors have a great range of treatments such as drugs, surgical operations, blood transfusions and organ transplants. But prevention is always better than treatment. Understanding how your body might become ill and how to keep it healthy is an important part of this prevention.

△ A week or two after the cold, you may have forgotten all about it.

PREVENTION FACTS

• Besides infections and allergies, there are several other types of health problems. Better prevention is possible in most of them.

• Injuries are a major health problem, especially in children and young people. Injuries range from a tiny cut in the skin to broken bones and crushed organs. Extra care and better safety could prevent many injuries.

• In some illnesses, various parts of the body become worn-out or no longer work properly. Take care not to overuse or strain your body with energetic sports or other activities.

• The exact causes of many cancers are not known. But doctors are discovering more links between cancers and features in our

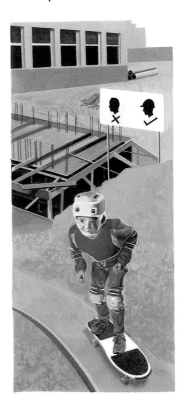

surroundings, such as polluting chemicals and harmful rays.

Things to do

KEEPING CLEAN

Good hygiene is an important part of preventing illness. Many germs are spread by touch, especially on your hands. Washing your hands well, with soap and warm water, helps to stop germs and illnesses from spreading. You should always wash your hands after using the bathroom, before meals, and before handling food. To see how dirty your hands get in a day, wash your hands as normal, but put a waterproof plastic bag over one hand each time you wash, to keep the soap and water from cleaning it. See how dirty it looks at the end of the day, compared to the clean hand! Remember to eat with your clean hand!

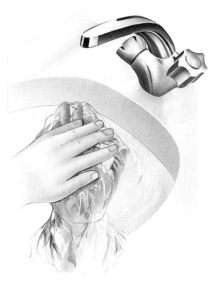

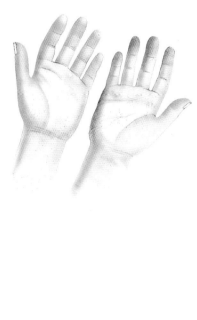

CATCHING GERMS

"Coughs and sneezes spread diseases." When you have an infection like a cold, your coughs and sneezes spread germs into the air, which could infect other people. Catch your sneezes in a tissue or handkerchief. If your nose is stuffed, blow it and get rid of the germs, rather than sniffing and keeping them. Blow gently into a paper tissue. Don't pinch either of your nostrils too tightly, though. This could blow mucus and germs into your ear and cause an ear infection.

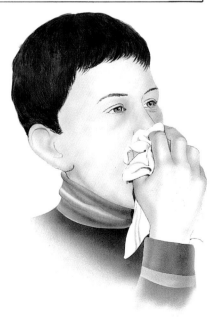

28

HIDDEN DIRT

Germs are so small that they get almost everywhere. Look at your fingernails. Are they really clean? Ask a grown-up to help you remove any dirt from under them with a nail file. If you can, look at this dirt under a magnifying glass or small microscope. Each tiny speck, almost too small to see, could be coated with hundreds of germs!

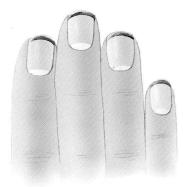

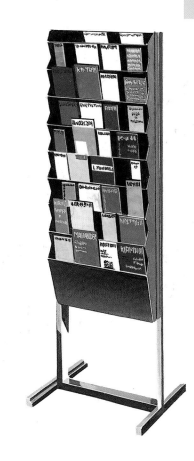

FIND OUT MORE

Visit your local doctor's office, clinic, hospital, dentist, optician and druggist, to see if they have free leaflets about health and illness. How many can you find about preventing illness? Do you ever have leaflets at school, for example, about head lice? Perhaps you have been to a talk or to a demonstration about first aid or road safety. All of this information will help you to find out more about how your body works, and how to prevent or treat illness.

HELPFUL BACTERIA AND FUNGI

Not all germs cause illness. Many are harmless to humans, and some are even helpful. Bacteria in your intestines help your digestive system to extract nourishment from your food. Similarly, not all fungi-type germs are harmful. In fact one type of fungus, called penicillium, was found to make a substance that killed many types of bacteria germs. This substance is the well-known antibiotic drug, penicillin.

Glossary

Allergy When the body reacts defensively to a harmless substance, such as grass pollen grains.

Antibodies Substances made by white blood cells, which attack germs. Antibodies are smaller than the tiniest germs.

Germ A tiny living thing that causes illness. Individual germs can be seen only under a powerful microscope. The main types of germs are bacteria viruses and fungi.

Hormone A natural body chemical made by an endocrine gland, which is released into the blood and affects certain parts of the body.

Hygiene Keeping the body clean and free from dirt and germs. Hygiene can also apply to clothes, food, and anything else that comes into contact with the body.

Hyperthermia When the body's temperature rises dangerously high, possibly damaging its internal temperature control system.

Hypothermia When the body's temperature falls dangerously low, possibly damaging its internal temperature control system.

Immune Being protected against or resistant to a certain infection. The germs are killed off by the body's inner defenses before they can multiply and cause illness.

Infection When germs get into the body and multiply, causing illness.

Lymph A pale fluid that flows slowly through a network of tubes in the body.

Lymphocyte A type of white blood cell that makes antibodies.

Mucus A sticky body fluid. It helps to protect delicate body surfaces such as the inside linings of the nose, windpipe and lungs.

Nasal cavity The hole behind your nose, and above your mouth. It opens into the throat at the back.

Red blood cells Doughnut-shaped cells floating in the blood, which carry oxygen around the body.

Symptoms The features of an illness that you notice, such as a headache or runny nose. The pattern of symptoms and how they change helps to identify the illness.

White blood cells Almost transparent cells found in the blood, lymph and other body parts. They can change shape and move, and they help to clean the blood and fight disease.

Resources

National Health Information Clearinghouse
P.O. Box 1133, Washington, D.C. 20013-1133, (800) 336-4797
(Phone or write to this clearinghouse for specific health information which concerns you.)

United States Government Printing Office
Superintendent of Documents
Washington D.C. 20402
(Request information on how to order free pamphlets on health-related issues.)

BOOKS TO READ

The Respiratory System by Mary Kittredge
New York; Chelsea House, 1989

Germs Make Me Sick: A Health Handbook for Kids by Parnell Donahue and Helen Capellaro
New York; Knopf, 1975

How Did We Find Out About Germs? by Issac Asimov
New York; Walker & Co., 1973

Your Immune System by Alan E. Nourse, M.D.
New York; Franklin Watts, 1989

Index

abdomen 19
allergies 26, 27, 30
anemia 15, 24
antibodies 21, 22, 30
asthma 26
athlete's foot 9

bacteria 9, 29, 30
blood 5, 12, 13, 14, 15, 16, 17, 21
bone marrow 17, 18, 19
bones 17, 18, 27
brain 6

cancers 26, 27
cells 12, 13, 14, 17
cerebellum 6
chicken pox 9, 20
cilia 23
coughing 8, 11, 28
diphtheria 9, 21
dysentery 9

ear infections 28
epidemic 5
eyes 4, 8

fever 5, 6, 7, 9, 24
flu see influenza
fungi 9, 30

germ-fighting cells 12, 13, 14, 16
German measles 21
germs 4, 6-7, 9, 16, 21, 22, 23, 28, 29, 30
glands 20, 30
goose bumps 8
gum disease 5

hay fever 26
headache 8, 24, 31
heart 13, 20, 22
heart disease 26
hygiene 28-29, 30
hypothalamus 6
hypothermia 7, 30

immune system 20-21, 30
immunization 21, 26
influenza 5
injuries 27
iron 19

lungs 22, 23, 24
lymph 16, 18, 21, 30
lymph system 12-13, 14, 19, 20
lymphocytes 18, 19, 20, 21, 30

malaria 5
measles 4, 9
medicine 11, 24, 26
mucus 4, 10, 11, 23, 24, 30

nose 4, 8, 10, 11, 14, 23, 24, 30, 31
nutrients 12

oxygen 14, 15, 31

plasma 14, 15
platelets 15
pneumonia 4
polio 21
protozoans 9
pus 16

red blood cells 14, 15, 16, 18, 19, 24, 31
ringworm 9
rubella 21

scarlet fever 9
schistosomiasis 25
shivering 6, 8
sickle-cells 15
skin 4, 26
sleeping sickness 25
smallpox 26
sneezing 8, 11, 28
sore throats 5, 24
spleen 19
sweating 6, 8
swollen glands 13
symptoms 8, 14, 24, 31

tear fluid 4
temperature 6, 7, 8, 9, 24, 30
tetanus 21
thermometer 6, 7
throat 10, 11, 14, 23, 24, 28, 30
thymus gland 20
tuberculosis 21

vaccine 21
viruses 9, 30
vitamins 24

white blood cells 14, 15, 16, 17, 18, 19, 20, 21, 30, 31
whooping cough 9, 21

x-ray 22